Khadija Sonda MOALLA
Nozha TOUMI
Rim SMAOUI

# Imaging cerebral venous thrombosis

Khadija Sonda MOALLA
Nozha TOUMI
Rim SMAOUI

# Imaging cerebral venous thrombosis

ScienciaScripts

**Imprint**



Cover image: www.ingimage.com

This book is a translation from the original published under ISBN 978-620-6-72611-1.

Publisher:
Sciencia Scripts
is a trademark of
Dodo Books Indian Ocean Ltd. and OmniScriptum S.R.L publishing group

120 High Road, East Finchley, London, N2 9ED, United Kingdom
Str. Armeneasca 28/1, office 1, Chisinau MD-2012, Republic of Moldova, Europe
Managing Directors: Ieva Konstantinova, Victoria Ursu
info@omniscriptum.com

Printed at: see last page
**ISBN: 978-620-8-53158-4**

## Contents

## List of abbreviations

- **MR** Angio-MRI
- **DS** Digital Subtraction Angiography
- **Flai** MRI sequence corresponding to the T2/recovery sequence by fluid-attenuated inversion.
- **cMR** Cerebral Magnetic Resonance Imaging
- **ISCVT** International Study on Cerebral Vein and Dural Sinus
- **S** Cavernous sinus
- **SP** Without injection of contrast medium
- **S** Sigmoid sinus
- **SS** Inferior sagittal sinus
- **SS** Superior sagittal sinus
- **S** Transverse sinus
- **C** brain computed tomography
- **T** Endovascular treatment
- **CV** Cerebral venous thrombosis
- **C** Cortical vein

# INTRODUCTION

Thanks to advances in imaging technology, cerebral venous thrombosis (CVT) is now an increasingly frequent pathology, with a favorable outcome when anticoagulant therapy is initiated in good time. However, the clinical picture is still highly polymorphous, and often not very suggestive, particularly at the beginning of its course.

The resulting therapeutic urgency requires imaging-based confirmation of the diagnosis. Cerebral angiography has long been considered the gold standard for the diagnosis of CVT(1) . Over the years, however, it has been replaced by non-invasive neuroimaging techniques (multi-bar CT and cMRI). Thanks to their higher resolution, these examinations make it possible to diagnose stroke at an early stage, guide the etiological diagnosis, monitor the disease and assess the prognosis .(2,3)

# CEREBRAL IMAGING

### *1. Cerebral venous angioscan*

CT without and with iodinated PDC injection at venous time is the examination of first choice due to its availability and rapid access. However, according to data from a recently published review, CT scans may be normal in 4 to 25% of cases, particularly when the clinical picture describes isolated signs of HTIC . [71,2]

#### 1.1 Direct signs

- **On injection-free sections**, certain direct signs are suggestive of CVT. The hyperdense triangle sign and the chord sign were observed in 26.6% and 31.6% of cases respectively . (4,5)

These signs appear during the first week, after which the spontaneous density of fresh blood gradually decreases. They are not very specific and may be falsely found in normal vessels with slow flow, in dehydrated patients and in cases of polycythemia .(2)

- **On sections with injection**, CVT is reflected by a defect in the enhancement of one or more venous structures, producing the "empty delta" or "empty triangle" sign.

In fact, it is the most specific CT sign of CVT. It is associated with a good sensitivity value ranging from 75% to 100%, in line with our results .(6)

However, this sign may be absent in the first 05 days because of possible contrast from the thrombus in the process of being organized or non-opacification of the sinus wall due to collateral circulation that has not yet developed. developed(7) . Similarly, a CVT may go undetected due to sub-optimal iodine injection time for exploration of the venous system . (8)

However, this examination can be fraught with interpretation difficulties, mainly anatomical in nature, leading to false positives such as sinus hypoplasia, asymmetric sinus drainage, Pacchioni granulations and the presence of an intrasinusal septum .(9)

On the other hand, the diagnostic performance of CT scans is less good for the diagnosis of cortical vein thrombosis, and does not allow its visualization in all cases when it is performed .(3)

The direct signs (dense triangle sign; string sign; empty delta sign) are illustrated in figures 1, 2 and 3 respectively.

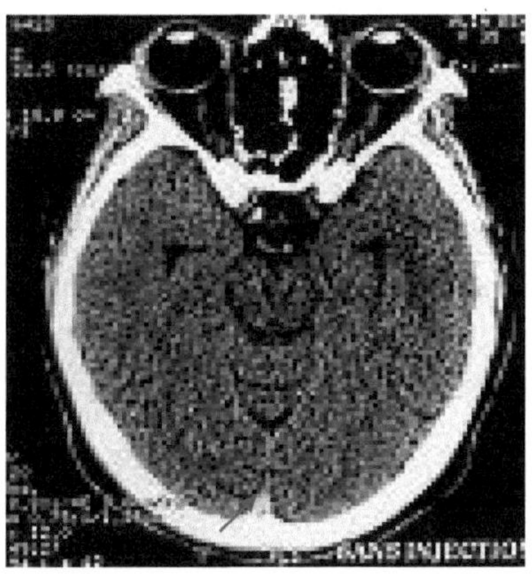

***Figure 1:*** ***SPC CT in axial section showing spontaneous hyperdensity of the sagittal sinus (= dense triangle sign)***

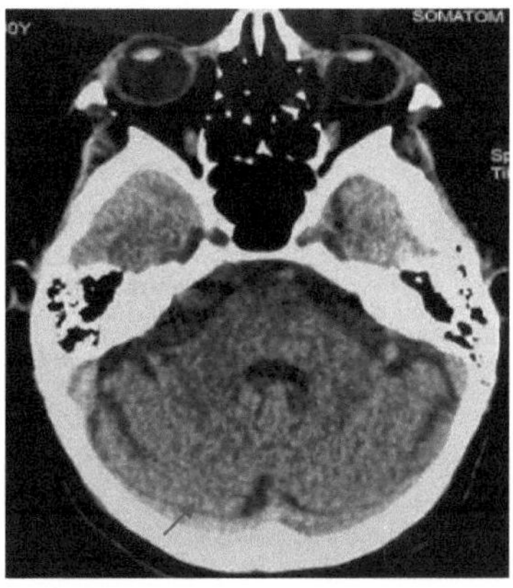


***Figure 2:*** ***SPC CT axial section showing spontaneous hyperdensity of the right lateral sinus (=string sign)***

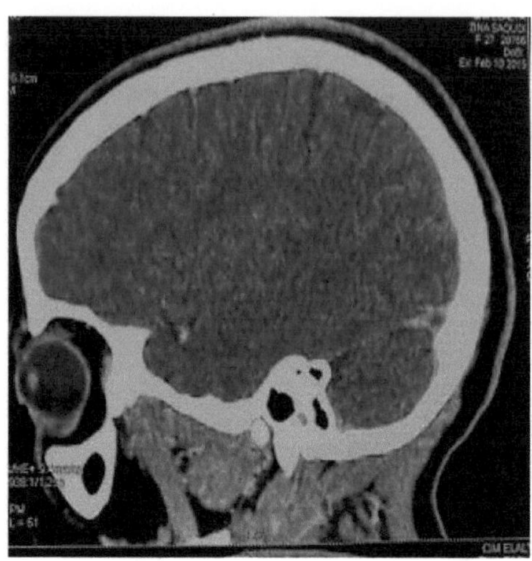

***Figure 3:*** ***CT scan with PDC injection, sagittal reconstruction illustrating a defect in SSS opacification (= empty delta sign).***

**1.2 Indirect signs**

Several indirect signs can be observed during a CVT:

- **On non-injected sections**, foci of venous infarction can be seen, usually bilateral, with or without a haemorrhagic component. The hemorrhagic component may be petechial or in the form of a true hematoma linked to a rupture of the blood-brain barrier(4) . The frequency of hemorrhagic infarction ranged from 39.2% to 77.7%(10–12) . Ischemic venous infarction is less frequent .(10–12)

  Other indirect signs may be promising, such as meningeal hemorrhage and/or subdural hematoma(13) . These signs are explained by increased retrograde pressure due to blockage of the cerebral venous system . (14,15)

Diffuse cerebral edema with compression of the ventricular system (appearance of small ventricles) could also suggest CVT (2%).

- **On PDC-injected sections**, abnormal contrast can be seen in the cerebral scythe and cerebellar tent. This is secondary to the development of "parietal" shunts in the dural wall .(4)

  Despite the multiplicity of direct and indirect signs, a normal cerebral venous angioscanner should not rule out the diagnosis of CVT, and should justify the use of cMRI.

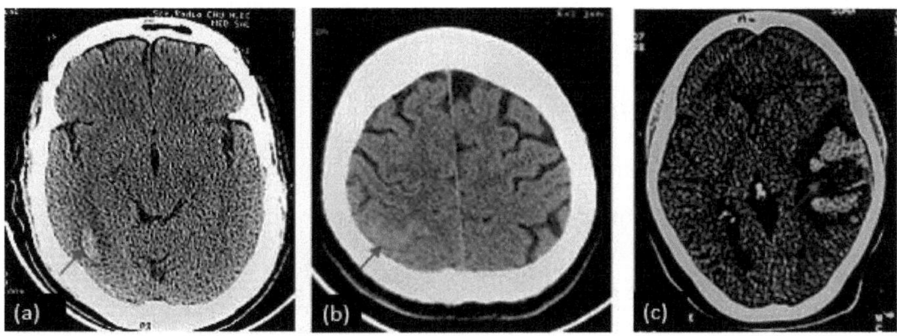


***Figure 4:** CT scan without injection of contrast axial slices illustrating indirect signs of CVT*

**a.** Spontaneous right temporal subcortical hyperdensity surrounded by edema in connection with thrombosis of the homolateral transverse sinus.

**b.** Spontaneous hyperdensity in the cortical sulci of the right parietal lobe revealing thrombosis of a cortical vein.

**c.** Left temporal cortico-subcortical oedemato-hemorrhagic patch exerting a mass effect on the homolateral lateral ventricle, reflecting venous softening with hemorrhagic transformation linked to thrombosis of the left lateral sinus.

### *2. Brain MRI*

cMRI is the reference examination for the diagnosis of a CVT, with an excellent sensitivity value of close to 100%(16) . It enables the thrombus to be visualized, its extent and impact on the cerebral parenchyma to be assessed, its evolution to be monitored and, in some cases, the pathology involved to be identified.

cMRI has been shown to be more sensitive than CT for the early detection of thrombus (including cortical vein thrombosis), minimal parenchymal lesions and cerebral edema .(17)

#### 2.1. Direct signs

Intraluminal thrombus appears in frank hyposignal independently of thrombus age on T2* sequence . (18)

This is because hemoglobin degradation products (oxyhemoglobin, deoxyhemoglobin, methemoglobin, ferritin and hemosiderin) shorten the T2 of the thrombus, resulting in a hypointense T2* signal.

Several studies have suggested the value of this sequence compared with other T1, T2 and Flair sequences in the diagnosis of CVT. Interpretation of these morphological sequences remains closely dependent on the evolution of the thrombus signal over time:

- In the acute phase (< 5 days), MRI may be falsely negative due to the appearance of thrombus in T1 isosignal and T2 hyposignal or T1 and T2 hyposignal, due to the presence of deoxyhemoglobin in intact red blood cells(18) . According to Favrole et al and Bergui et al, only 10 to 30% of thrombi are visualized at this stage . (19,20)

However, at this stage, a thrombus may not even be visualized on the T2* sequence. In this situation, MRA after injection of Gadolinium can overcome these difficulties. It can show an endoluminal lacuna, a defect in the enhancement of a dura mater sinus or cerebral vein, or the equivalent of the "empty delta" sign.

Gadolinium injection is contraindicated in cases of pregnancy, breast-feeding, allergy, renal insufficiency or history of renal transplantation. 2D time-of-flight (2D-TOF) MRA sequences with arterial flow saturation and MIP reconstructions are useful because they show a lack of visualization of the thrombosed sinus, contrasting with the intense hyper-signal of permeable veins. This sign is even clearer when sinus occlusion is complete . (2)

Partial thrombosis, on the other hand, may go undetected. On the other hand, certain pitfalls related to technical artifacts for time-of-flight MRA and/or anatomical variants sometimes lead to false positives, such as hypoplasia or agenesis of the transverse sinus (more frequent on the left and often associated with a small posterior torn hole), and Pacchioni granulations (signal close to that of CSF) .(21)

- In the subacute phase (day 5-15), the thrombus appears as a T1 and T2 hypersignal due to the conversion of deoxyhemoglobin to methemoglobin within the thrombus. This is the characteristic appearance according to Crassard et al and Lich et al .(13,18)
- In the chronic phase (>15 days), thrombus hypersignal decreases progressively(13) . The thrombus typically presents as T1 isosignal and T2 hyper/isosignal. However, thrombus signal can be significantly variable at this stage .(18)

In order to improve the diagnostic performance of cMRI in thrombus detection, particularly in contentious cases, a joint interpretation of the different sequences is recommended, notably the T2*- T13D GADO and 2D-TOF sequences.

According to recent studies, the diffusion sequence is playing an increasingly important role in the diagnosis of CVT. It can be useful for thrombus visualization, especially in patients requiring rapid exploration (e.g.: agitated state ), showing a frank hypersignal. According to recent studies, this hypersignal occurs in 30% of cases and is associated with a lower rate of recanalization under treatment [30].

However, exact dating of the age of the thrombus seems difficult to establish in the absence of parallelism between the onset of clinical signs and thrombus formation. This is explained by the fact that clinical manifestations may be delayed in relation to thrombus formation, unlike in arterial stroke [77].

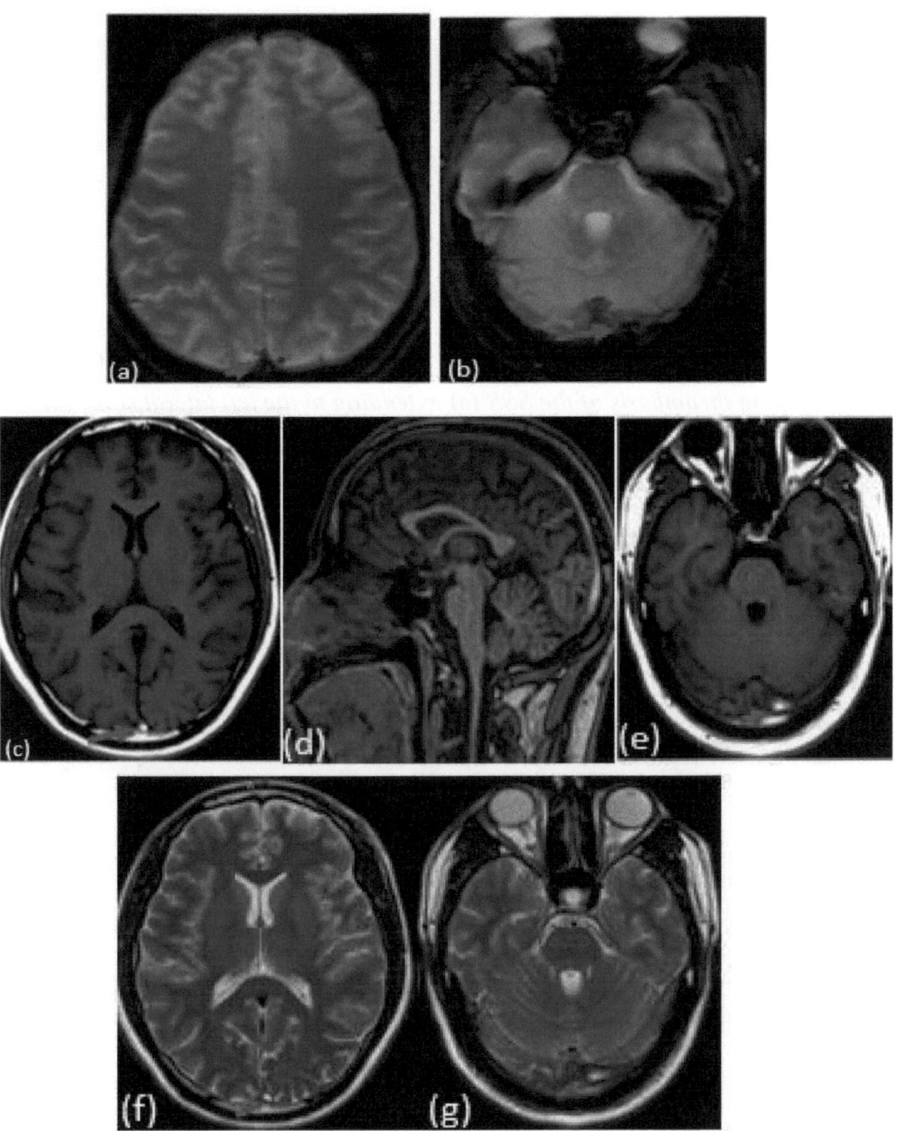


***<u>Figure 5:</u> Axial slice cMRI showing subacute thrombus of the SSS and STG, T2* hyposignal (a and b) T1 hypersignal (c, d and e) and T2 hypersignal (f, g)***

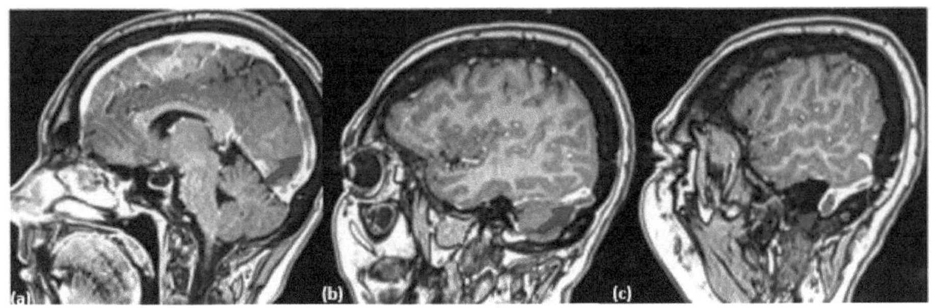


***<u>Figure 6:</u> cMRI with T1 3D GADO sequence in sagittal reconstructions showing thrombosis of the SSS (a) extending to the left lateral sinus (b) and homolateral jugular vein (c)***

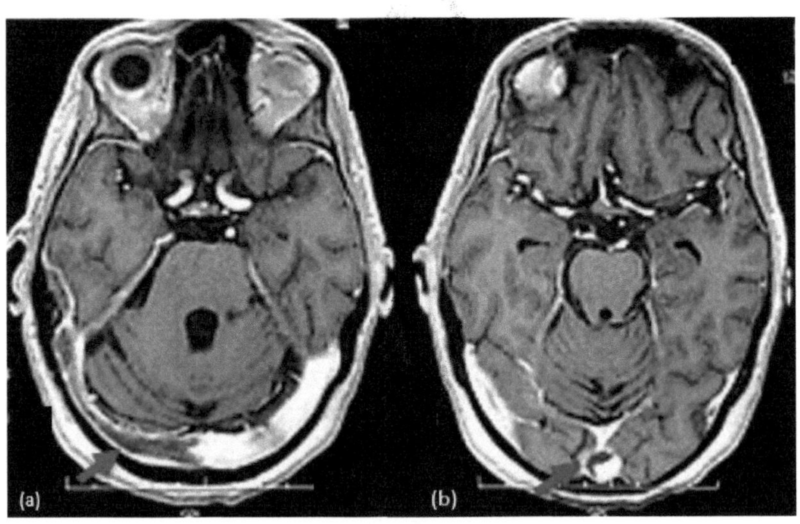


***<u>Figure 7:</u> cMRI with T1 3D GADO sequence in axial slices showing an enhancement defect of the right transverse sinus (a) with heterogeneous contrast of the SSS (b) "empty delta sign" .***

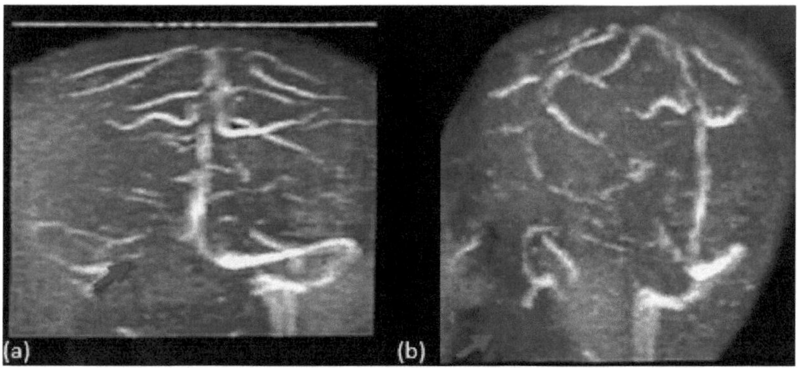


***Figure 8:* 2D-TOF sequences in coronal (a) and sagittal (b) planes, showing a visualization defect of the right lateral sinus and jugular vein, contrasting with good visualization of the contralateral venous system.**

**2.2. Indirect signs**

They are essentially represented by venous softening, the appearance of which varies greatly according to the stage of evolution(9) . In the early stage, vasogenic edema is seen at the cortical and subcortical levels, with T1 hyposignal and T2 hypersignal without restriction of ADC. In a second stage, intracellular edema appears, evidenced by a clear restriction of diffusion. At a later stage, a rupture of the blood-brain barrier with the appearance of hemorrhagic foci .(4) These signs are aspecific, but their diagnosis has been facilitated by the demonstration of a signal anomaly in thrombosed sinuses .(4)

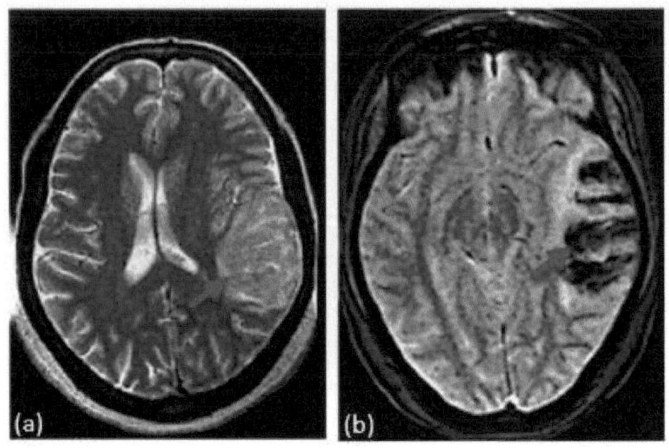


***Figure 9:* cMRI with T2 (a) and T2* (b) sequences in axial sections showing a left temporoparietal lobar hematoma .**

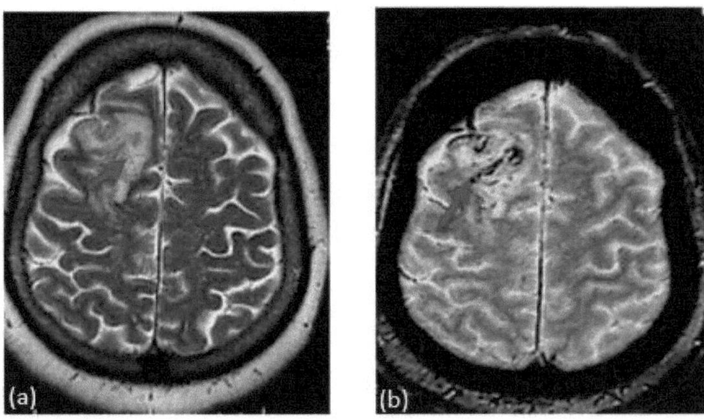


***Figure 10:* cMRI T2 (a) and T2* (b) axial slices showing hemorrhage at the bottom of a cortical groove surrounded by edema, indicating thrombosis of a cortical vein .**

According to the latest recommendations, thanks to diffusion imaging, cMRI provides prognostic value by assessing the extent of lesions and, above all, differentiates between vasogenic edema (increased ADC value/reversible lesions) and cytotoxic edema (decreased ADC value/irreversible lesions) (Figure 11) .(19)

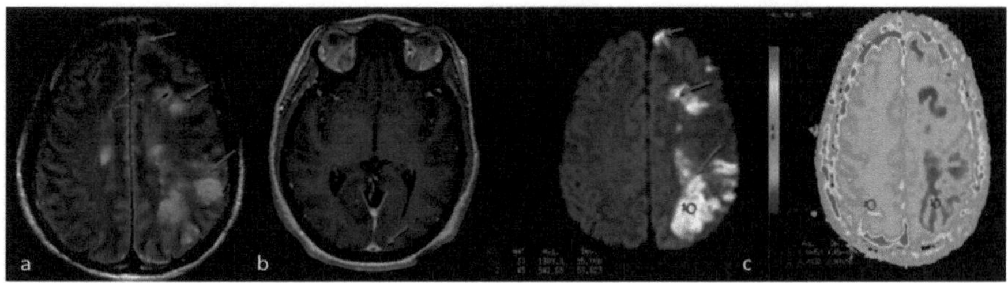


***<u>Figure 11:</u> Brain MRI with Flair (a), T1 3D Gado (b) and diffusion (c) sequences showing a hyerpsignal in left fronto-parietal patches with clear restriction of the DW reflecting cytotoxic oedema related to venous infarction linked to thrombosis of the SLS. (11)***

**2.3 Etiological signs**

In some patients, cMRI provides etiological guidance by showing a locoregional infectious or tumoral cause or post-traumatic lesions . (4)

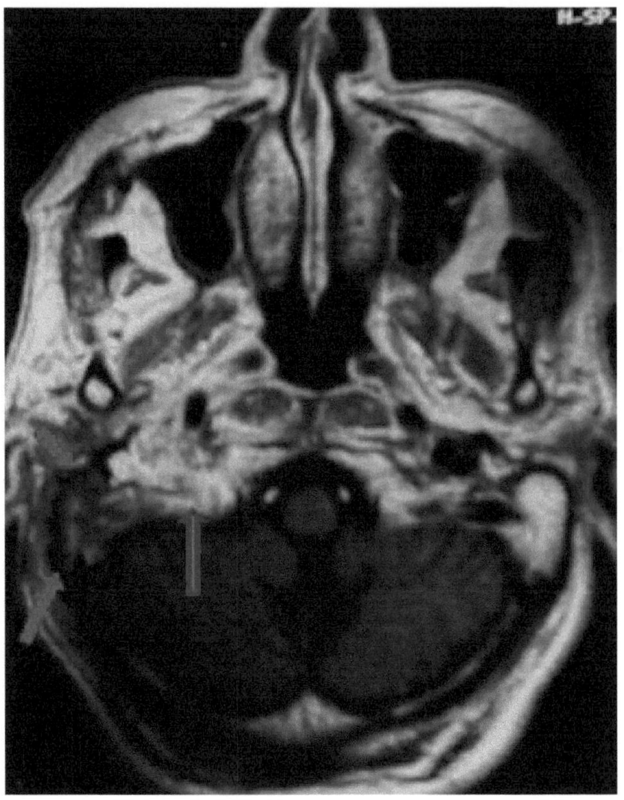

***Figure 12:** cMRI shows malignant otitis externa complicated by CVT of the right sigmoid sinus extending to the VJD (red arrows): Flair hypersignal of the medial part of the right ACE extended to the jugular foramen and homolateral parapharyngeal space (blue arrow).*

### *3. Radiological particularities depending on the site of thrombosis and clinico-radiological correlations*

Thrombosis most often affects veins and sinuses simultaneously, and frequently spreads from one sinus to another, from a sinus to a cerebral vein, or vice versa(10,22–24) . Apart from locoregional causes, where the location of the clot is often close to the causative condition, CVT can affect any venous structure.

It is clear that SSS, ST and SS are the most frequently affected in the literature (Table I).

***<u>Table II :</u> Review of literature data on***

***on the site of CVT***

| | *Multiple* | *SSS* | *STG* | *STD* | *SS* | *SC* | *VC* |
|---|---|---|---|---|---|---|---|
| **ISCVT (n=624)** (22) | _ | 62% | 44,7% | 41,2% | NP | 1,3% | 17,1% |
| **VENOST (n=1144)** (23) | 51,8% | 38,9% | NP | NP | 39,8% | 1,7% | 3,7% |
| **Touati (n=160)**(10) | 68,6% | 65% | 38,1% | 45,6% | G : 35%<br>D : 37,5% | 1,8% | 8,7% |
| **Yedaes (n=41)** (25) | 43% | 52% | 30% | 34% | 21% | 2% | 5% |
| **Alami (n=62)** (4) | 34% | 52% | 45% | 45% | NP | 5% | 2% |
| **FPCCVT (n=231)**(24) | 68,3% | 48,3% | 33,8% | 47,6 | G : 26,8%<br>D: 40,3% | 0,4% | 7,3% |

SSS: superior sagittal sinus; STG: left transverse sinus; STD: right transverse sinus; SS: sigmoid sinus; SC: cavernous sinus; VC: cortical vein; L: left; R: right

Clearly, inter-individual variation in cerebral venous anatomy and the frequent association of thrombosis in several sinuses and veins make precise clinico-topographic correlation difficult [3]. Certain thrombosed venous structures are associated with particular radioclinic forms:

### 3.1 Thrombosis of the superior sagittal sinus

The most frequently encountered signs are headache and HTIC syndrome. EC is often associated with thrombosis of the SSS. .(26)
Venous softening can occur in the para-sagittal regions of the fronto-parietal and parieto-occipital and in the basal regions of the temporo-occipital, thus explaining the clinical polymorphism of damage to this structure . (1)

### 3.2. Thrombosis of a cortical vein

Thrombosis of a cortical vein is rare. It occurs preferentially in hemispheric veins of the frontal and parietal regions(27) . According to Liu et al and Ahn et al, it is often associated with thrombosis of another sinus . (28,29)
According to the literature, clinical manifestations are dominated by headache, motor deficit, and CE(30) . In our series, in line with the literature, MRI is more sensitive in detecting thrombosis than CT .(8,26,31)
The identification of an edematous and/or hemorrhagic cortico-subcortical focus prompts us to look for certain suggestive signs, such as the "rope" sign on uninjected CT, a T2* hypo signal tracing the path of a cortical vein (Figure 13) and the "rail" sign after injection of PDC . (27)
In certain contentious cases, and when there is a strong clinical suspicion, cerebral angiography may be justified.

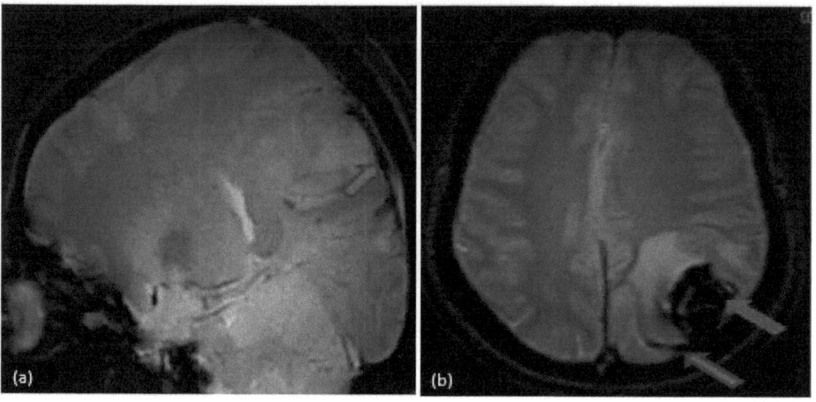


***Figure 13:*** ***T2* sequence in sagittal oblique (a) and axial (b) sections showing hyposignal (rope sign) of a cortical vein (blue arrow) with a left parietal hematoma (red arrow) .***

### 3.3. Thrombosis of the cavernous sinus

Thrombosis of the cavernous sinus is rarely described in the literature. It should be suspected in the presence of a variable combination of the following signs: chemosis, painful ophthalmoplegia, exophthalmos, palpebral edema, cranial nerve damage (II, III, V1, V2, VI)(32) . Isolated VI involvement is plausible. Initially unilateral symptoms may become bilateral if thrombosis extends to the contralateral cavernous sinus or other dural sinuses (Figure 14) .(32)

The diagnosis can be made by CT scan, which shows a lack of opacification, heterogeneous enhancement of the cavernous lodge, enlargement with bulging of the lateral border, more or less associated with other indirect orbital signs (exophthalmos, densification of intraorbital fat, dilatation of the ophthalmic vein) .(33–35)

MRI shows an enlarged cavernous lodge, isointense with gray matter in T1, and abnormally hyperintense and heterogeneous in T2 acquired in this case, in axial and especially coronal slices. After injection of gadolinium, the thrombosed part of the cavernous lodge shows a lack of enhancement, contrasting with intense enhancement of the non-thrombosed part and the meningeal walls .(35)

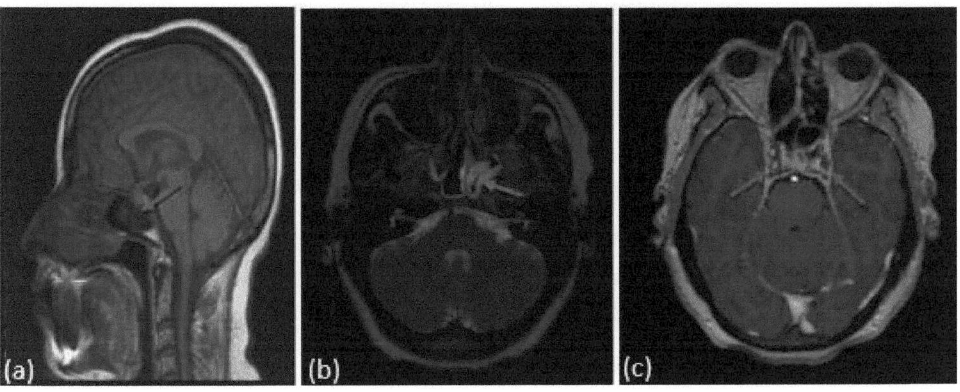


***Figure 14:** T1 sagittal section (a) and T2 (b) and T1 3D GADO (c) axial sections showing bilateral cavernous sinus thrombosis (red arrows) secondary to sphenoidal sinusitis.*

### 3.4. Thrombosis of the deep venous system

CVTs involving the deep venous system are uncommon, with respective values of 11% in the ISCVT study . (22)

They affect the right sinus, the ampulla of Galen, the internal cerebral veins and Rosenthal's basilar veins, and most often result in bilateral, but asymmetrical, edematous and/or hemorrhagic lesions in the thalamo-capsular and sometimes lenticulo-capsulo-caudate areas and in the deep white matter (Figure 15). Lesions may extend into the midbrain and upper part of the vermis and cerebellar hemispheres(36,37) . This radiological presentation may pose a differential diagnosis with a glial tumor, arterial ischemia, Gayet-Wernicke, global hypoxia or carbon monoxide intoxication. In this situation, in addition to the clinical context, T1 3D GADO sequences can be used to verify the permeability of the deep venous network, thanks to multi-planar reconstructions in the sagittal plane. Similarly, venous angioscanner, with the advent of the new generations, is proving very useful in confirming or refuting the hypothesis of thrombosis of the deep venous system .(3)

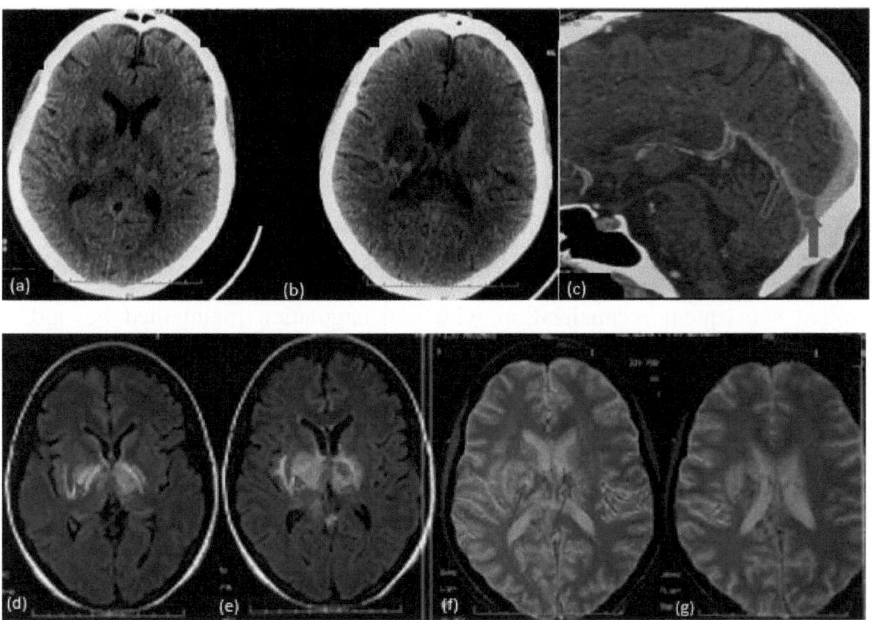


***Figure 15:* CT and MRI appearance of deep vein thrombosis deep vein thrombosis**

PDC-free cTd in axial slices (a, b): bilateral capsulothalamic hypodensities, splenium of corpus callosum and right periventricular white matter. CT reconstructions in sagittal plane at venous time (c) showing opacification defect of torcular (large solid arrow), right sinus (large empty arrow) and internal cerebral veins (small solid arrow).

cMRI showing a bithalamic Flair hypersignal (d,e) extended to the capsulo-lenticular region (d) with hemorrhagic remodeling better visible on T2* sequences (f,g).

### *4. Radiological evolution*

According to a multicenter observational study that included 551 patients with confirmed CVT who received anticoagulation therapy with systematic radiological monitoring from 30 days(38) , male gender was shown to be associated with no or partial repermeabilization. Similarly, according to this study(38) , the majority of recanalizations occurred early in the course, suggesting limited subsequent recanalization with anticoagulation maintained beyond 3 months. In the same context, Herweh et al assessed the percentage of recanalization as a function of time in 99 patients and concluded that recanalization is most often observed within 3 to 6 months of diagnosis(39) . In rare cases, recanalization may occur beyond 6 months. They therefore suggested that the decision to continue anticoagulant therapy beyond 12 months should not be based on the degree of recanalization, but on the risk of thrombosis recurrence and the presence of a persistent pro-thrombotic state.

In addition, the recrudescence or persistence of HTIC signs after a CVT should suggest dural venous stenosis, in addition to recurrence. CE-3D-MPRAGE and 3D-T1-SPACE sequences have proved useful in differentiating between CVT and dural sinus stenosis.

The presence of symptomatic dural sinus stenosis should prompt venous pressure measurement by retrograde phlebography. TE (stenting) may be considered in patients with a significantly increased pressure gradient between the proximal and distal segments of the stenosis .(40)

# CONCLUSION

A good understanding of the radiological semiology of DVT will enable a positive diagnosis to be made, so that anti-coagulant treatment can be started early, with the aim of improving prognosis.

We emphasize that MRI combined with venous magnetic resonance angiography (MRA) is the reference examination for the diagnosis of CVT, with good sensitivities and specificities, as well as its repercussions on the cerebral parenchyma. However, venous angioscanner remains the first-line examination, given its availability, and is initially used to rule out differential diagnoses.

# REFERENCES

1. Dmytriw AA, Song JSA, Yu E, Poon CS. Cerebral venous thrombosis: state of the art diagnosis and management. Neuroradiology. july 2018;60(7):669-85.

2. Sadik JC, Jianu DC, Sadik R, Purcell Y, Novaes N, Saragoussi E, et al. Imaging of Cerebral Venous Thrombosis. Life (Basel). August 10, 2022;12(8):1215.

3. Carletti F, Vilela P, Jäger HR. Imaging Approach to Venous Sinus Thrombosis. Radiol Clin North Am. May 2023;61(3):501-19.

4. Alami B, Boujraf S, Quenum L, Oudrhiri A, Alaoui Lamrani MY, Haloua M, et al. Cerebral venous thrombosis: clinico-radiological aspects, about a series of 62 cases. JMV-Journal de Médecine Vasculaire. Dec 2019;44(6):387-99.

5. Rodallec MH, Krainik A, Feydy A, Hélias A, Colombani JM, Jullès MC, et al. Cerebral Venous Thrombosis and Multidetector CT Angiography: Tips and Tricks. RadioGraphics. Oct 2006;26(suppl_1):S5-18.

6. Ghoneim A, Straiton J, Pollard C, Macdonald K, Jampana R. Imaging of cerebral venous thrombosis. Clin Radiol. Apr 2020;75(4):254-64.

7. Shinohara Y, Yoshitoshi M, Yoshii F. Appearance and disappearance of empty delta sign in superior sagittal sinus thrombosis. Stroke. 1986;17(6):1282-4.

8. Arquizan C. Cerebral thrombophlebitis: clinical aspects, diagnosis and treatment. Réanimation. June 2001;10(4):383-91.

9. Saposnik G, Barinagarrementeria F, Brown RD, Bushnell CD, Cucchiara B, Cushman M, et al. Diagnosis and management of cerebral venous thrombosis: a statement for healthcare professionals from the American Heart Association/American Stroke Association. Stroke. Apr 2011;42(4):1158-92.

10. Touati Nahla. Epidemiological, clinical and radiological study of cerebral venous thrombosis: About 160 cases.

11. Mahdi Frikha. Imaging of cerebral thrombophlebitis: Retrospective study about 104 cases.

12. Yii IYL, Mitchell PJ, Dowling RJ, Yan B. Imaging predictors of clinical deterioration in cerebral venous thrombosis. Journal of Clinical Neuroscience. nov 2012;19(11):1525-9.

13. Crassard I, Bousser MG. Cerebral venous thrombosis: an update. La Revue de Médecine Interne. Feb 1, 2006;27(2):117-24.

14. Oliveira IM, Duarte JÁ, Dalaqua M, Jarry VM, Pereira FV, Reis F. Cerebral venous thrombosis: imaging patterns. Radiol Bras. 2022;55(1):54-61.

15. Hassan A, Ahmad B, Ahmed Z, Al-Quliti KW. Acute subarachnoid hemorrhage. Neurosciences (Riyadh). jan 2015;20(1):61-4.

16. Dormont D, Anxionnat R, Evrard S, Louaille C, Chiras J, Marsault C. MRI in cerebral venous thrombosis. J Neuroradiol. Apr 1994;21(2):81-99.

17. Van Dam LF, Van Walderveen MAA, Kroft LJM, Kruyt ND, Wermer MJH, Van Osch MJP, et al. Current imaging modalities for diagnosing cerebral vein thrombosis - A critical review. Thrombosis Research. May 2020;189:132-9.

18. Leach JL, Fortuna RB, Jones BV, Gaskill-Shipley MF. Imaging of Cerebral Venous Thrombosis: Current Techniques, Spectrum of Findings, and Diagnostic Pitfalls. RadioGraphics. Oct 2006;26(suppl_1):S19-41.

19. Favrole P, Guichard JP, Crassard I, Bousser MG, Chabriat H. Diffusion-weighted imaging of intravascular clots in cerebral venous thrombosis. Stroke. Jan 2004;35(1):99-103.

20. Bergui M, Bradac GB. Clinical picture of patients with cerebral venous thrombosis and patterns of dural sinus involvement. Cerebrovasc Dis. 2003;16(3):211-6.

21. Poon CS, Chang JK, Swarnkar A, Johnson MH, Wasenko J. Radiologic diagnosis of cerebral venous thrombosis: pictorial review. AJR Am J Roentgenol. Dec 2007;189(6 Suppl):S64-75.

22. Ferro JM, Canhão P, Stam J, Bousser MG, Barinagarrementeria F, ISCVT Investigators. Prognosis of cerebral vein and dural sinus thrombosis: results of the International Study on Cerebral Vein and Dural Sinus Thrombosis (ISCVT). Stroke. March 2004;35(3):664-70.

23. Duman T, Uluduz D, Midi I, Bektas H, Kablan Y, Goksel BK, et al. A Multicenter Study of 1144 Patients with Cerebral Venous Thrombosis: The VENOST Study. Journal of Stroke and Cerebrovascular Diseases. August 1, 2017;26(8):1848-57.

24. A TB, I C, L D, M BG, R M, E RB, et al. Cerebral Venous Thrombosis: Clinical, Radiological, Biological, and Etiological Characteristics of a French Prospective Cohort (FPCCVT)-Comparison With ISCVT Cohort. Frontiers in neurology 2021, vol. 12, p. 753110.

25. Yedeas MD. Cerebral venous thrombosis: a clinical, etiological, radiological and prognostic study.

26. Ulivi L, Squitieri M, Cohen H, Cowley P, Werring DJ. Cerebral venous thrombosis: a practical guide. Pract Neurol. Oct 2020;20(5):356-67.

27. Boukobza M, Crassard I, Bousser MG, Chabriat H. MR Imaging Features of Isolated Cortical Vein Thrombosis: Diagnosis and Follow-Up. AJNR Am J Neuroradiol. Feb 2009;30(2):344-8.

28. Liu KC, Bhatti MT, Chen JJ, Fairbanks AM, Foroozan R, McClelland CM, et al. Presentation and Progression of Papilledema in Cerebral Venous Sinus Thrombosis. Am J Ophthalmol. May 2020;213:1-8.

29. Ahn TB, Roh JK. A case of cortical vein thrombosis with the cord sign. Arch Neurol. Sept 2003;60(9):1314-6.

30. Song L xi, Lu H yu, Chang C kang, Li X, Zhang Z. Cerebral venous and sinus thrombosis in a patient with acute promyelocytic leukemia during all-trans retinoic acid induction treatment. Blood Coagul Fibrinolysis. oct 2014;25(7):773-6.

31. Song S ying, Lan D, Wu X qin, Meng R. The clinical characteristic, diagnosis, treatment, and prognosis of cerebral cortical vein thrombosis: a systematic review of 325 cases. J Thromb Thrombolysis. Apr 2021;51(3):734-40.

32. Levine SR, Twyman RE, Gilman S. The role of anticoagulation in cavernous sinus thrombosis. Neurology. Apr 1988;38(4):517-22.

33. Munawar K, Nayak G, Fatterpekar GM, Sen C, Zagzag D, Zan E, et al. Cavernous sinus lesions. Clin Imaging. Dec 2020;68:71-89.

34. Idiculla PS, Gurala D, Palanisamy M, Vijayakumar R, Dhandapani S, Nagarajan E. Cerebral Venous Thrombosis: A Comprehensive Review. Eur Neurol. 2020;83(4):369-79.

35. Nagi S, Kaddour C, Jeribi R, Marrakchi-Turki Z, Ben Yahmed A, Skandrani L, et al [Cavernous sinus thrombosis secondary to sinusitis]. J Radiol. June 2008;89(6):803-5.

36. Herrmann KA, Sporer B, Yousry TA. Thrombosis of the internal cerebral vein associated with transient unilateral thalamic edema: a case report and review of the literature. AJNR Am J Neuroradiol. Sept 2004;25(8):1351-5.

37. Benabdeljlil M, El Alaoui Faris M, Kissani N, Aïdi S, Laaouina Z, Jiddane M, et al [Neuropsychological disorders after bithalamic infarction caused by deep venous thrombosis]. Rev Neurol (Paris). Jan 2001;157(1):62-7.

38. Salehi Omran S, Shu L, Chang A, Parikh NS, Zubair AS, Simpkins AN, et al. Timing and Predictors of Recanalization After Anticoagulation in Cerebral Venous Thrombosis. J Stroke. May 2023;25(2):291-8.

39. Herweh C, Griebe M, Geisbüsch C, Szabo K, Neumaier-Probst E, Hennerici MG, et al. Frequency and temporal profile of recanalization after cerebral vein and sinus thrombosis. Euro J of Neurology. Apr 2016;23(4):681-7.

40. Y F, J Y, H C, J Z, J D, D M, et al. Chinese Stroke Association guidelines for clinical management of cerebrovascular disorders: executive summary and 2019 update of clinical management of cerebral venous sinus thrombosis. Stroke and vascular neurology, 2020, vol. 5, no. 2.

# APPENDICES

# <u>Appendix 1:</u> Anatomy of the cerebral venous system

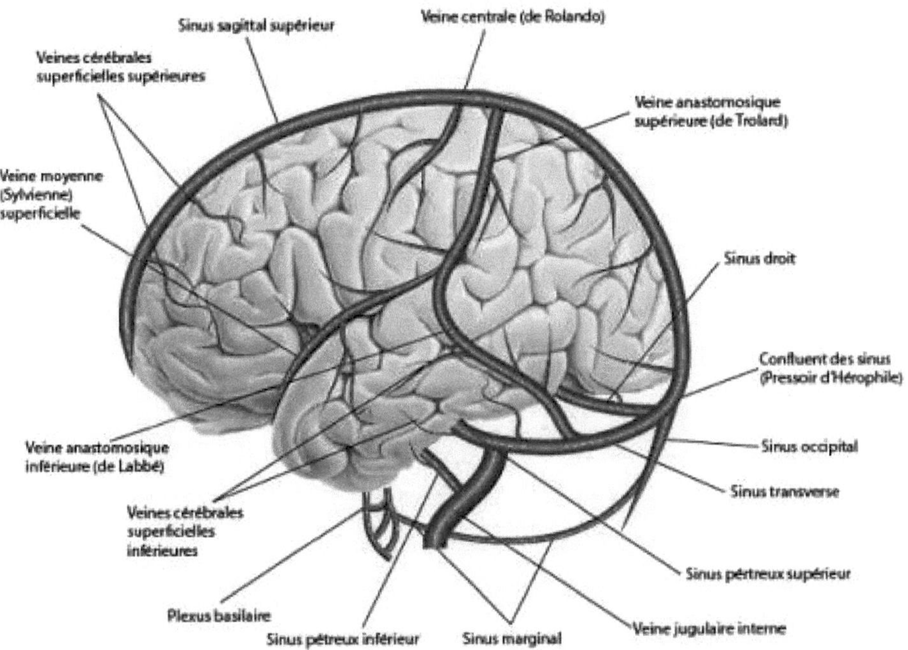


***Fig. 1: Venous structures on the lateral surface of the brain***

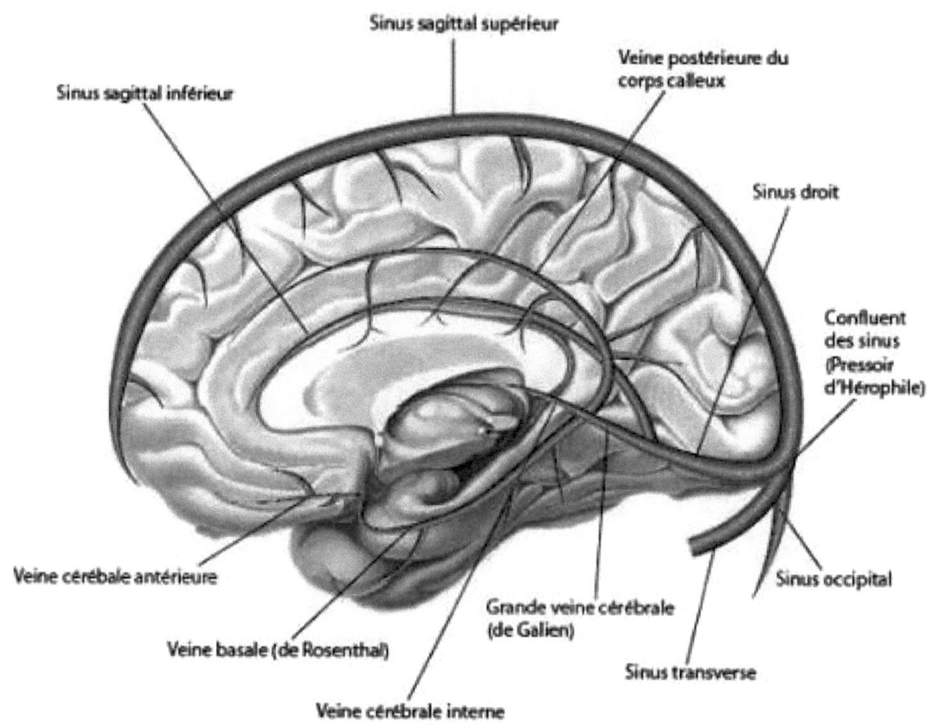


***Fig. 2: Venous structures on the medial side of the brain***

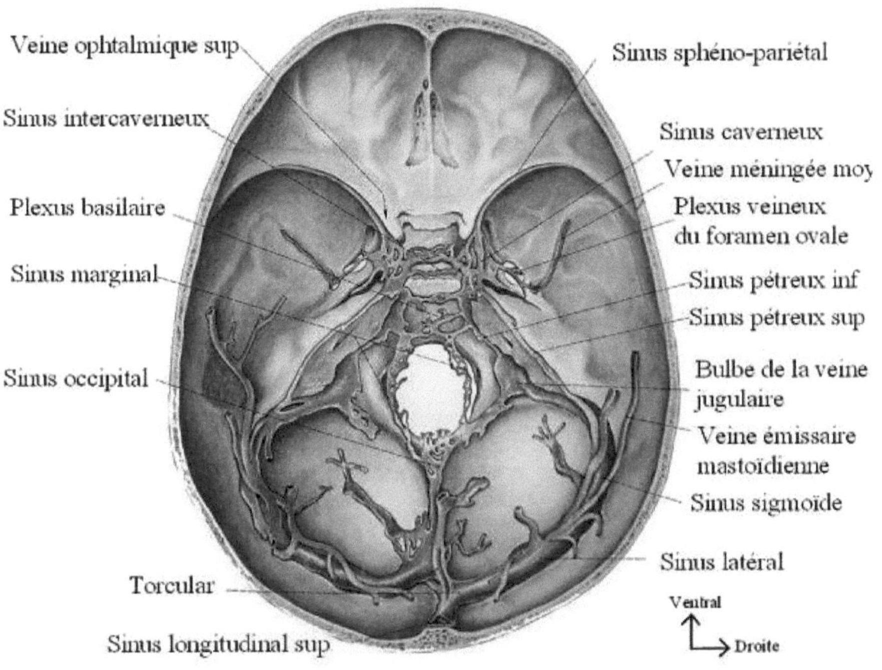


***Fig. 3: Endocranial view of skull base venous drainage***

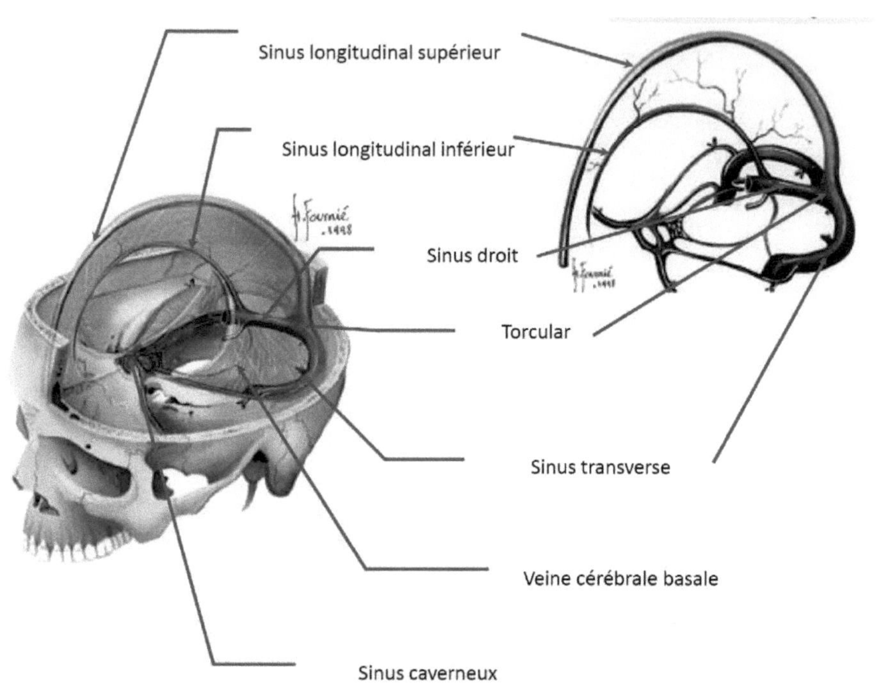


***Fig.4: 3D diagram of the cerebral venous system***

The venous blood of the brain is drained by three networks of cerebral veins: the superficial (cortical) veins, the deep veins and the veins of the posterior fossa.

These veins drain into the dural venous sinuses, which are in turn collected by the jugular veins (Fig. 1).

The small cortical veins drain blood from the cerebral parenchyma through the subarachnoid and subdural space. The two internal cerebral veins and the two basal veins of Rosenthal lead blood from deep cerebral structures, such as the thalamus and the trunk ganglia, to the great vein of Galien (Fig. 2).

The odd-numbered superior sagittal sinus (SSS) drains most of the cortex. It joins the right sinus at the level of the torcular (sinus confluence or Herophilus press) (Fig. 2).

The lateral sinuses (LS), which are even, consist of two segments: the transverse sinus and the sigmoid sinus. The size of these sinuses is often unequal: the largest (usually the right) is continuous with the SSS, while the other receives blood from the right sinus. In 20% of cases, there is partial or total agenesis of a transverse sinus.

The odd-shaped inferior longitudinal sinus (inferior sagittal sinus) drains the inner surface of the middle hemispheres and the corpus callosum.

The odd right sinus is the confluence of Galien's vein and the inferior longitudinal sinus. It drains into a transverse sinus (usually the left) or into the torcular.

The paired cavernous sinuses are crossed by nerve (III, IV, V1, V2, sympathetic plexus) and vascular (internal carotid) structures. They drain mainly the orbits and the superficial middle cerebral vein. Blood flows to the lateral sinus and jugular vein via the petrous sinuses. The two cavernous sinuses are anastomosing, which explains why thrombosis is often bilateral (Fig. 3).

## APPENDIX 2: Pathophysiology of DVT

Although the conditions that can lead to cerebral venous thrombosis (CVT) are extremely varied, three main pathophysiological mechanisms are involved: disorders of hemostasis (leading to a prothrombotic state), venous stasis and parietal abnormalities (Virchow triad).

The cerebral impact of CVTs is uncertain, and depends on the existence of bypass grafts, and the site and extent of thrombosis.

Thrombosis of the sinuses initially leads to an increase in venous and capillary pressure, resulting in rupture of the blood-brain barrier and the onset of vasogenic edema. At the same time, if pressures continue to rise, a reduction in tissue perfusion leads to the appearance of ischemic lesions and cytotoxic edema.

Thrombosis also leads to reduced resorption of cerebrospinal fluid by Pacchioni's granulations, helping to increase venous pressures and the appearance of parenchymal changes. Hyperpressure rupture of arterial and venous capillaries can lead to hemorrhagic lesions. Cerebral lesions can range from simple edema, usually reversible, to parenchymal hematoma involving both cortex and subcortical white matter.

Bleeding may be parenchymal and/or occur in the subarachnoid, subdural spaces and ventricular cavities. Parenchymal lesions may be distant from the site of occlusion, and thrombosis of a median sinus may result in bilateral, paramedian cerebral lesions without arterial systematization.

Vasogenic edema reflects a rupture of the blood-brain barrier and plasma extravasation into the interstitial environment. It is reversible with effective treatment of venous occlusion. Cytotoxic edema, a consequence of ischemia, reflects irreversible lesions.

## APPENDIX 3

## Direct and indirect signs of CVT on imaging

| Direct signs | Indirect signs |
| --- | --- |
| • Dense triangle sign (clot in sinus on NECT)<br>• Cord sign (thrombosed cerebral vein on NECT). MRI equivalent: thrombosed vein seen on gradient echo or susceptibility weighted images or rarely other sequences<br>• Empty delta sign (clot as filling defect within the sinuses on CTV/CE-MRV)<br>• Replacement of normal dark flow void with clot on MRI | • Cerebral edema with elevated or mixed diffusion characteristics<br>• Hemorrhagic infarction<br>• Subarachnoid hemorrhage<br>• Rarely, subdural hemorrhage |

NECT : CT scan without contrast injection, CTV: venous angioscanner, CE-MRV: venous MRA,
MRI: magnetic resonance imaging

## Appendix 4

# Evolution of thrombus signal on sequences

## MRI sequences

Evolution of MRI signal intensity caused by venous thrombus.

| | Haemoglobin degradation product | T1 | T2 & FLAIR |
|---|---|---|---|
| <5 days | Deoxyhaemoglobin | Iso/hypointense to brain tissue | Iso/hypointense to brain tissue |
| 6 days to 2 weeks | Methaemoglobin | Hyperintense | Hyperintense |
| >2 weeks | (Fibrosis/recanalisation) | Variable | variable |

FLAIR, fluid attenuation inversion recovery.

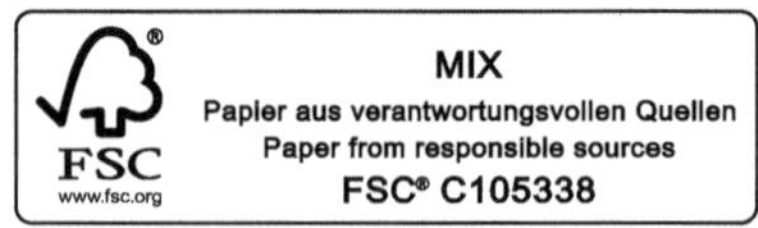


Printed by Books on Demand GmbH, Norderstedt / Germany